The 10-Second Diet

A Technique You Can Master in Less Time Than It Takes to Read the Cover of the Book

MernaLyn

ISBN: 1-4392-7282-4
ISBN-13: 9781439272824

Lillian

Enjoy Life
'10 seconds'
at a
time

Merralyn
2014

Mom, if you saw me walking down the street and you didn't know me...

Table of Contents

Chapter 1
You Can Do It

Why don't diets work? First of all, they can be too difficult to understand and follow. Secondly, it takes too long to see the results. Thirdly, you can feel deprived of foods you enjoy, which negatively affects your mood and disposition. The **10-Second Diet** changes all that! This is a revolutionary new approach to a very old problem: losing weight. The **10-Second Diet** enlightens you to the only way anything can be successful—by stopping and thinking before acting, and using the most powerful aspect you have as a person, your brain. This is why it works, and this is how you can learn a technique to attain your personal self-fulfillment.

As we begin, let's look at **10** things this book is NOT:

1. This book is not hard to read.
2. This book is not full of confusing terms or concepts; it is easy to understand.
3. This book is not expensive, but it is as valuable as the price you put on your health and well-being.
4. This book is not about only one aspect of your life, losing weight. It is about a technique you can master to apply to *all* aspects of your life to become the best person you can be.
5. This book is not a cookbook. You do not need to eat special foods or follow specific recipes.
6. This book is not long. Who has time to read another two- to four-hundred-plus-page diet book?
7. This book is not your conscience. It does not condemn your choices nor condone your habits.
8. This book is not an excuse to ignore what you know is best for your good health.

9. This book is not a fad; its concepts are real and accurate, and will endure for all time.
10. Lastly, this book is not a one-time read. It is a good refresher and a lifelong handbook, and will be fun to reread whenever you like.

Now that you know ten things this book is NOT about, let's see what this book IS about. You are about to discover a philosophy that will enable you to control your attitude about dieting and eating, and allow you to enjoy your life with food as a part of living—not as the *reason* for living.

It is easier to conceptualize doing something rather than actually *doing* it. It is much more comfortable to think, *Tomorrow I'll start my new diet. I'll eat smartly, I'll eat less, and I'll exercise more. It will be easier to begin tomorrow.* Does this sound familiar? Well, guess what? Today is all those "tomorrows" you have been appeasing yourself with. If you did not start the day "dieting," you may feel it really doesn't make any sense to begin a new routine in the middle of the afternoon or late in the day. But what if I tell you with certainty that you can begin your new life-eating routine RIGHT NOW? It doesn't matter if you've eaten a dozen chocolate chip cookies, or overindulged in the morning-doughnuts-in-the-office coffee break. It doesn't matter if it's nine in the morning or nine at night. You can start right now. Why? Because this is the only "now" you can live. So why not start now?

This is the no-diet diet. If you learn and follow the simple technique, you will never need to stress over foods or diets again.

If you feel skeptical, that is understandable. This may be a new concept you are not accustomed to. However, it will work for you if you give it a try. You will be amazed at how simple it is. Isn't it nice that, finally, something so simple works so effectively? You do not need months or weeks to notice an improvement in your life. It is effective in only **10** seconds!

Let's say this book will help you through the first few minutes of your new routine. After all, it will take a little time for you to read this. But that's just not enough. It is one thing to assimilate the concepts when you are not hungry or craving anything. (Providing you can differentiate between the two; but what if you can't? We'll discuss differentiation later in the book.) What if that hunger presents itself and you can't think of anything but that brownie you brought home from the bakery calling to you from the kitchen counter? (Well, actually, it's the backup brownie you bought when you bought the one you had to eat right away while it was still warm—what luck that you stopped at the bakery right after they were taken out of the oven! Hmm).

What now? This may not be what you think you would be reading right now, but go and get the brownie. I'll wait. Are you back? OK, I didn't say "eat" the brownie. I said "get" the brownie. Now it's you, the brownie...and this book.

Put the brownie in front of you. That's all. Don't eat it, just look at it. Smell the brownie, touch it. Bring all your senses into the same place and time. This might seem existential, but why not try it? You bought this book. Let's see how this works. (It does!)

Now, count to **10** slowly and deliberately. If you are totally fixated on the brownie, then think about it. It is a baked good. That's it. It does not control you. YOU control you. Now you can do one of many things. You can put the brownie back in the bag. You can continue to stare at it. You can devour it in one unsatisfying swallow and berate yourself afterward. You can take a *tiny* taste, a little bite, and truly TASTE it. You can count to **10** and decide if you want to make the first change in your life or not. YOU CAN DO THIS. The brownie is nothing but flour, sugar, eggs, chocolate, vanilla, and salt. It does not control you. YOU control you. You have volition. You have ability. You have power over what you do. If you choose to take a taste, then do so, but really taste it, perhaps as if it were the first time. Feel the texture as you pick it up and while it is in your mouth. You are your own judge, but do not be your own jury. Do not admonish yourself. Be kind and understanding. This is just the first time you are trying something new. After your first little bite, put the brownie away. Come back and read what to do next. How are you doing? If you have taken the (little) bite you wanted to, have put away the brownie, and are now back to reading, then you have done great! This might be the first time you have ever thought so much about a bite to eat and that's fine. It's about time you really thought about food in this perspective. And it's just the beginning.

It is important to keep in mind why you are eating. You have the choice and thought process to assess your impulses every time you think about eating something. Although the initial response may be to pop the first thing you see into your mouth, this is the perfect time to STOP and THINK. Why are you eating what you are about to eat? Are you truly hungry or eating because of an impulsive habit? Confronting yourself with these questions each and every time you are about to eat will create a new part of your routine, until these questions become rote and you will ask them rhetorically and answer them naturally.

More doesn't necessarily equate to better. More is just more. STOP and THINK. Do I really need more, or have I satiated my craving and more will not benefit me?

Putting unnecessary calories into your body in no way helps you to overcome loneliness, sadness, or boredom. Think about this: nothing tastes as good as feeling good about yourself feels. All it does is ultimately put you further into a detrimental state, because when the eating attack is over you will have to deal with your self-loathing, sense of guilt, and criticism of yourself. You know you do not need that; it is not the way to feel good about yourself. Stuffing senseless calories into your body will not take away any negative feelings you are experiencing. You need to STOP and THINK and do something good for yourself; something that does not have to do with putting food in your mouth. It bears repeating: nothing tastes as good as feeling good about yourself feels.

It's time for a small, easy remedy to stop yourself from overeating...

Here's a great little trick for you to try. When you are done eating, or before you have completely finished, walk away from the food and go brush your teeth. If you are not at home, carry a travel-sized bottle of mouthwash with you and go to the restroom and use it. If that's not possible, or if you feel uncomfortable doing this in a public facility, just pop a mint into your mouth. The minty freshness tells your mind you are done eating and gives it a time-out to really evaluate whether or not you want/need to eat any more. Who wouldn't want to trade hundreds of calories for a tiny one-and-a-half-calorie (or less if it's sugarless!) refreshing end to a meal?

MY OWN WORDS

1. What are my thoughts and feelings about what I just read?
2. What will help me "connect" to myself and enhance my mind-body-psyche fulfillment?
3. How can I best use what I just read to my benefit and make it my own?

MY OWN WORDS continued...

MY OWN WORDS continued...

MY OWN WORDS continued...

MY OWN WORDS continued...

Chapter 2
Stop & Think

Whatever it is you are about to eat, think about it. Think carefully, for at least **10** seconds, before you decide you will eat it. How much simpler could this be? Take the time to think about why you want to eat whatever it is you are contemplating eating. Again, no matter what it is, condition yourself to really *think* about it. What benefit will it be? What detriment? Just THINK before your first bite.

OK, it's you and the brownie again. (The brownie is used only as an example; you can substitute any food item you may be craving.) Put the brownie on the plate in front of you and look at it as you did before. Let's say you have now decided to eat the brownie. If the term "my" brownie is used, you have already commanded ownership of it and it is a lot harder to give up the idea that it is not "yours." Isolate the food as nonpersonal.

Food is to nourish the body and improve or maintain health as well as to enjoy. None of these factors involve the intake of copious amounts to satisfy those conditions. Here is where the **10-Second Diet** again comes into practice. Think of cutting your portion into **10** equal pieces. No matter what is on the plate, physically cut it into **10** equal pieces. Now, take one of the **10** pieces. Look at it, smell it—REALLY look at and smell it. Notice its color and visual texture. Lastly, put it in your mouth. Before you start to chew, be aware of how it feels. Then, bite down on it and notice how the flavor and texture changes. Chew it a minimum of **10** times. If it requires more, do so. Do not rush your eating experience.

After you swallow, stop. Think about what you just ate. Wait **10** seconds before having another bite, if you want more. This is the eating experience.

We live in an accelerated world, one where we require our fast food to rival our high-speed Internet. It seems as though everything must be accomplished quickly. However, this does not necessarily equate to efficiency or quality, especially in the case of nutrition, nourishing not only our bodies but our entire being. We are complex organisms reliant on a harmonious relationship of the physical, mental, and psychological. So often we ignore the harmony or lack cognizance of these three aspects. There is a balance to nature and we are part of that balance. To maintain each individual's unique balance, all three factors must be considered.

How do we consider the three aspects of physical, mental, and psychological in relation to food? A simple approach (which this book strives for!) is to consider:

Physical: Am I really hungry? Do I feel hunger pangs?

Mental: What will this food do to benefit my body and help it perform to its own potential? Why am I choosing to eat this particular food? Is it the right time to eat? What is the caloric value of what I am about to ingest?

Psychological: Why am I eating now? Why am I choosing to eat this particular food? These questions have different answers here than when considered under the "Mental" section. ("Do I know when I am hungry or eating for other reasons?" will be discussed later in the book.)

One can no more separate the interrelatedness of these three aspects of life than one can separate threads woven together to make a sturdy piece of cloth. Without the substantial interweaving of all the threads, there would be a gaping hole, something flimsy and unsupportive. This is also true in our daily lives. So, how can a diet be effective if one of the major components is missing or being ignored? It can't. One must consider and evaluate all three aspects.

1) Physical: How much weight do I want to lose? I need to listen to my body and know when I am genuinely hungry.

2) Mental: I can configure the number of calories and determine how much I need to eat to balance against the amount of energy I expend in a day.

3) Psychological: I know I am not really hungry; why am I eating this now? What am I actually feeling? Am I depressed? Happy? Bored? What do I want to accomplish by eating this?

The **10** words below will help you accomplish your weight-loss goal and acknowledge your psychological aspect. These are the "definitive **10**":

I CAN DO THIS.
IT WILL WORK!
JUST **STOP**!
THINK!

It will take you just **10** seconds to say this, either to yourself or out loud. This will reinforce the confidence you need to accomplish your desire and redirect your focus, allowing your mind the immediate change of course it needs to stop what you are doing and get on the right track to lead you down your road of personal control.

Each of us is unique and special. To truly feel this we need to accept who we are and gain control over the aspects of ourselves we would like to change and improve. If this is in the area of weight control, then the key to unlocking the answer lies in our psychological selves. We need to have a combination of awareness, recognition, and assertion of the three aspects of every human being: physical, mental, and psychological.

We all know what willpower is and how hard it is to maintain, especially at the time it's needed the most. Instead, try strengthening your "won't power" by saying to yourself: "I won't eat that. I won't do that. I won't say that." By learning to refrain from immediately responding without forethought you will encourage the strength you have within. You are capable of doing this. Decide to do what is best for you after considering the possibilities presented to you at the moment. Choose not to do things that will impair your success along the path to your personal fulfillment. This will benefit you on your diet as well as your life path. This exemplifies the techniques essential for eating and living well.

The word "diet" has taken on a derogatory meaning. It has become synonymous with being deprived of foods that make one feel happy. "Diet" does not refer only to food. According to Webster's dictionary, a diet is: a habitual course of living. There can be a monetary diet, which we may refer to as a budget. Not spending more than one earns would be the equivalent of not overeating food. A work diet is a balance of work to play, without which one becomes a workaholic. A humanitarian diet is a diet rich in kindness and positive gestures to humanity. Doing and thinking more about other people would provide a healthier diet for both sides. A diet does not have to be an undesirable state you do not look forward to being in, yet find yourself perpetually and frustratingly inhabiting.

Each person has the capability of doing the right, humane, decent thing. Each person has personal choice. There are some who choose to be completely oblivious to the fact that their actions affect other people. There may be a lack of awareness, no social conscience, or an inability to understand or empathize when relating to another human being. How does this lack of personal responsibility correlate to the **10-Second Diet**? It would be most beneficial to think of the consequences of one's actions; however, this would require an ability to rationally understand that there is a link between an action and a subsequent result. This may be a difficult process for some to cultivate. Therefore, if one can learn to STOP before continuing an undesirable action, this may be a start. Through repetition, almost anyone can create a learned response to STOP. STOP—before self-destructively eating that next bite. The time to STOP is when you find yourself in a situation when you know better and are inclined to do something anyway, without regard for the consequences. STOP before inflicting harm to oneself or someone else. One more high-fat, calorie-laden bite will not necessarily kill you, or do irreversible injury to you, but one bite after another after another might. Just STOP and THINK about it.

This may all sound too easy. That's not just the point; it's the solution. Life presents enough challenges without making it more difficult. Try to keep life simple. Does this seem idealistic? Let's look at the concept of "idealistic," with "ideal" being defined as: a conception of something in its perfection; a standard of perfection or excellence. Wouldn't it be perfect if you didn't have to diet to attain the weight you want? Wouldn't it be perfect if you were truly content with your life? One has to identify and nurture both internal and external facets of being to do this. The three aspects and their correlation to one another cannot be ignored. To expect success in dieting by reading the latest diet fad, measuring and consuming just the correct amount of food, and exercising proportionally, yet ignoring the pleasure and comfort of eating, is to deny an entire one-third of the human makeup. It is this psychological aspect that gives us the emotional satisfaction required, which volumes of consumption cannot measure up to.

The human being is a complex mechanism that is continually evolving. It seems that in this society, we have been able to accept the physical aspects of humanity, but that is the base part of it. This is what we can see and touch. We understand that the mental and physical parts can be in sync and that there is a connection. However, we also need to embrace the psychological part of humanity, for this part is the motivating factor that implicitly directs the mind to engage the body. It is when these three essential components interrelate that we can fully function as members of humankind.

It is time to stop genuflecting to superficiality. Now is the time to begin appreciating the unique quality of individuality. It is essential to learn to accept and respect the features, coloring, and physical aspects of each person and not judge unfairly or one-dimensionally by only considering the external packaging. You find a truer happiness when seeing and feeling the beauty that comes from accepting and loving yourself and others just the way you or they are.

There is so much emphasis on the physical. As a society, we need to elevate to a higher level and worship the mind as much as we seem to worship the body. The body is our vehicle through life. The mind is where our true self lies; it is our psyche that creates who we uniquely are. It is our subconscious as well as our coherent understanding and interpretation of our life experiences that create the person we project ourselves to be.

The mind is the substantial core where the germination of thought begins. It is the basic place where one's thoughts and ideas form, but the subconscious may be responsible for the way they form.

Babies aren't born with a how-to tag telling how best to nurture and raise them. We don't come with an instruction manual on how to live life. We are currently in a state of S.O.S.—Save Our Society! Nike says, "Just Do It." I say, "Just DON'T Do It until you STOP and THINK!"

MY OWN WORDS

1. What are my thoughts and feelings about what I just read?
2. What will help me "connect" to myself and enhance my mind-body-psyche fulfillment?
3. How can I best use what I just read to my benefit and make it my own?

MY OWN WORDS continued...

MY OWN WORDS continued...

Chapter 3
Keep It Easy

You may be wondering, why is it the **10-Second Diet?**
Not the Minute Diet or some other time element. Why **10?**
Have you ever heard that, when you are angry, before responding with something you may later regret you should
count to **10?** Have you ever wondered why? Counting to **10**
shifts the immediate focus of the brain. Those brief **10** seconds are enough to arrest the previously self-programmed
response and allow a break in thought processes. This is the
pause needed to reprogram and create the new response,
which is not only a new way to think of food and eating, but
will result in the success of any diet you choose and may
well eliminate the necessity for any other dieting program.
This concept can be applied to other aspects in life as well.
It is that immediate break in focus, that momentary diversion which creates an avenue to accept another thought
that previously would not have had a chance to arise. In this
case, it is the opportunity needed to reconsider whether or
not to ingest more calories. Those **10 seconds** create the
opening necessary to decide if you are really hungry or just
responding to what would ordinarily be a programmed reaction to continue eating because there is still food in front
of you.

Let's look further into the concept of "**10,**" which is an
ultimate definitive number. As Ben Schott, author of *Schott's
Original Miscellany* and the yearly almanac *Schott's Miscellany,* and contributing columnist to the op-ed pages of
The New York Times, states, "In biblical hermeneutics* the

number **10** represents the perfection and completeness of the divine order—as in the Ten Commandments."

*her·me·neu·tics (hûr'mə-nōō'tĭks)—the science of interpretation, esp. of the Scriptures.

There is a comfort, a completeness to the concept of "**10**." The number **10** is attainable.

When referring to ranking on a scale, we say, "What would you give the movie on a scale of one to **10**?" "How do you like my outfit on a scale of one to **10**?" Some people may want to be referred to as a "perfect **10**." To each his or her own "**10**." In other words, you can and should be your own "perfect **10**." It is a subjective grade. Yours can be a size 18, a size 2, or even a size **10**!

The number **10** has become a qualitative definitive in life.

The mind can more easily accept a simple concept than a complex one; therefore, there is a higher possibility of success when the technique is simple.

OK, how many of you want "easy"? Let's see a show of hands. (I know my hand is raised!) Well, the weight will not roll off just because you want it to, but something like that. How easy is it to just THINK? If the desire is there, the thoughts are there, and the motivation is there, then the success *can* be there.

One of the reasons diets fail is because they focus on only one aspect: the physical. We cannot disassociate one of our three aspects from the others and expect to have lasting success in any part of life, much less in dieting.

We tend not to take responsibility for the thing that influences us the most: our brain. Irrespective of any external stimuli, the brain has the ability to accept or reject an impetus. A thought may enter the mind, but what we choose to do with it is our own volition.

Most people are aware of their physical body and know they have a mind, but are less aware when it comes to realizing they have an entire psychological makeup. There are subconscious reasons one reacts the way one does. One has to become aware of the fact that one's reaction to anything originates subliminally. One thinks with the brain, but *feels* with the mind. Thoughts come from the brainwaves but are generated through experiences interpreted in the mind. All are an inseparable part of a human being. All three aspects must be realized, acknowledged, and nurtured, or it is like living as two-thirds of a person instead of incorporating the entire package and living as a whole human being.

An old saying is that the definition of "stupid" is doing the same thing again and again and expecting a different result. It takes months or years to try to rewire the effect life's experiences have on the psyche. To believe you can keep doing the same detrimental thing in your life and think it will mysteriously have a new outcome and suddenly improve your situation is wishful thinking. You must take a different and effective approach to losing weight, and the same is true for living life. There is a successful and expedient way to achieve your goal, whether in dieting or any other aspect of life, and the **10-Second Diet** technique shows you how!

You can't devour an entire piece of food without cutting it up into smaller "digestible" pieces. The same is true of understanding a new concept. You can best comprehend this by relating it once again to the three aspects previously referred to:

Physical: You can't scale an entire mountain with one large step, but you can take one small step at a time until you safely and securely reach the peak.

Mental: You may not be able to understand an entire math theory all at once, but breaking it down into smaller equations and understanding each one thoroughly allows the larger solution to become clear.

Psychological: First, just realizing there are deep-rooted aspects embedded in your mind that are motivating your responses is primary in moving forward in the direction of your goal.

It would be dishonest to claim that you will lose weight just by thinking. However, everything—EVERYTHING—begins as a thought, which may evolve into a thought process. Like links in a chain, one thought triggers another and another until you have a concept. You need to grasp a simple concept, one that works and will continue to work as you use it. Just like exercise, it does become easier. And when it starts out easy, how much easier can it get? Here again is your thought, which has already been put into a thought process and conceptualized (now that's easy!):

I CAN DO THIS.
IT WILL WORK!
JUST **STOP**!
THINK!

There you are. Easy. A simple mental diversion; a shift of focus. It takes just **10 seconds**. Just **10** little words, yet capable of creating a lifetime of change.

Saying "I CAN DO THIS" to yourself creates a positive, strong mental directive. "IT WILL WORK" reaffirms and solidifies the optimistic success of your attempt. "JUST STOP" arrests your thought process and refocuses your actions to enable you to redirect your THINKing.

Take control of yourself. You have the power; *it* does not have the power over you!

You have succeeded. You are master of your own **10** seconds!

Prior to this, with your unsuccessful attempts to diet, you may have had a feeling of powerlessness or hopelessness. But, as it is said, where there is life there is hope, just as where there is creative thought there is possibility—possibility to improve the life you have. There are those who mentally run away from their own emotions, people afraid of their feelings or thoughts of personal inadequacies. There are those who think that to "feel" is to be weak; really, it is the other way around. Those who can "feel" and accept their vulnerability are those who truly have the strength. Compassion, empathy, concern, love—all of these are human, sensitive feelings. Without acceptance and understanding of the human emotions, people can superficially float through life, without really submersing themselves in it, which is like carefully wading into the water and never actually diving in.

Human beings can be empty shells of existence if they eschew and underestimate the power of psychological-mindedness. Accept nothing but success. Anything else is simply not acceptable, agreeable, or allowable. NOTHING short of your own desired success will do. You must accept this. You must allow this. You must believe in and adhere to this. There is no other option, there is no other resolution. You must resolve this and this alone to be the result of your actions, as it is the only outcome of your desires. You will succeed, for there is no other option. It is a given. You must believe this with all your being. This is the way to your personal fulfillment. There is no other choice.

We live in an un-psychologically-minded society. There seems to be a pervasive fear of the unknown. People seem to be able to accept a physical affliction, and perhaps even a mental one, more readily than they could ever confront or accept a psychological implication, even if it infringes on their health. One thing we must learn and understand: everything that affects us is three-parted. There is the physical, the mental, and the psychological. Everything we do in life depends on the interaction of these factors. At times one may seem to be more dominant, but never are they totally independent of each other. Dieting is no different. Perhaps we have tried endless variations of calorie counting and portion control. We may have even been able to understand the relationship between planning our diet and adhering to it, and that with the introduction of exercise these things may produce the desired weight loss. Yes, it makes sense to realize that fewer calories taken in combined with physical exercise is a sensible way to lose weight. We do not always respond to sensible, however. Not to mention that most predominant of factors: how EASY it is for us. It is hard to get much easier than counting to **10,** don't you think?

There might be vulnerability and apprehension when one even considers the idea of confronting one's feelings—the psychological aspect of life. One can look in a mirror so readily and assess one's physiology, but not look inward to one's psyche. There have been references previously to "un-psychological-mindedness" in this book, but what exactly does this mean?

"Un-psychological-mindedness" means being un-aware of the fact that feelings and thoughts are interrelated to the human existence. It also means being impervious to others' feelings and thoughts, and to the idea that one's actions are precipitated by these very feelings and thoughts. The realization of this, along with incorporating and executing a mindful way of living, brings about a more psychologically minded and considerate world.

Wouldn't you love it if you could just close your eyes and wish to lose all the weight you wanted, and when you opened your eyes—*poof*—you **were** that ideal weight? Let's try it. Are you ready? OK. Eyes closed. Repeat after me: "I wish I were _____ pounds. I wish I were _____ pounds. I wish I were _____ pounds." Open your eyes. How did you do? Did you lose the weight? Of course, this didn't and won't work. If you have tried everything you thought possible to lose weight, then this book is for you. If you genuinely want to lose weight in as easy a way as possible, truly this book is for you.

The reason this works is because it is easy to understand and simple to execute.

People underestimate the power of the mind and the interrelatedness of the physical-mental-psychological relationship that constitutes a human being. I refer to this relationship as the "triune diet-y" (physical/mental/psychological). One aspect does not exist without the other two and all coexist in harmony together.

Let us look at this "triune diet-y" as, again, a brownie. A brownie has flour, cocoa, and eggs. If you were to try to construct a brownie without any one of these ingredients, you would be unsuccessful. If the flour were omitted, there would be no substance; without the eggs, there would be no cohesiveness; and without the luscious quality of the cocoa, there would be no sensuality.

You push yourself to work out (the physical), you watch your calories (the mental), and yet you ignore the catalyst to make the other two successful (the psychological). Most importantly, it is here where all things become possible.

We are a product of what we believe and what we believe in. If we believe it, it is true to us. If we believe something will work, it opens up our realm of possibility to allow us to work toward what we hope to accomplish coming to fruition. Therefore, to be successful in a weight-loss endeavor, we must first believe we *can* be successful, then find a way we believe will enable us to accomplish our personal fulfillment. This, of course, must be done with logical consideration. We will not accomplish weight loss if we only *believe* we can and do nothing physically and mentally to work toward it. By identifying a dieting concept that we find amenable to us and believing it to be compatible with our individual personality and character, it has a far greater chance of actually being successful for us and fulfilling our weight-loss goal.

For example, one cannot eat high-calorie, fat-laden foods and simply wish the calories away. This is not the *Wish Fulfillment Diet*, as it would be unfeasible and completely irrational to even entertain the thought that it would ever work. Again, everything in life reflects three things—physical, mental, and psychological—and the symbiosis that exists among them.

The logical reason that the **10-Second Diet** works is because stopping and shifting the focus in your brain alters your train of thought. You have complete control to just

STOP. It is completely within your realm NOT to EAT. You are in command of your brain, your thoughts, and your inner dialogue. It is within your control because you are the master of your mind. This is the success you seek and this is the way you will gain control over your impulses. You will succeed at mastering and controlling your responses just **10 seconds** at a time! This is an instant and gratifying result that you need to feel you have accomplished. Relish the feeling. It will prompt you to enjoy this personal fulfillment and continue your success in bite-sized pieces until you conquer what, at the beginning, seemed to be insurmountable, and achieve your goal.

MY OWN WORDS

1. What are my thoughts and feelings about what I just read?
2. What will help me "connect" to myself and enhance my mind-body-psyche fulfillment?
3. How can I best use what I just read to my benefit and make it my own?

Chapter 4
Keep Moving

Let's look at **10** Things to Do NOT to Eat:

1. Physically move away from the food after your **10** bites. Just get up and walk to a room without any food in it. There is a psychological response that triggers your desire to eat if you see, smell, or taste food. The type of food you respond to is a personal thing. It may reflect a happy experience from your past, and without realizing it, you feel that by eating the item again you will be transported to the warm and comforting feeling you had when you first encountered that food. If you understand this aspect and are aware that it may be the motivating factor behind your craving, it will help you to overcome eating for eating's sake. Realize that the food was one component of your experience and nothing you overeat can take you back in time to that exact situation. That was then; envelop yourself in the memory, not the food.

2. Get out of the house. Take a walk. Just put one foot in front of the other and MOVE! If you can't go outside, start walking in the house; go to a different floor, run up and down the stairs—it's good exercise and it physically removes you from being next to the food. Make a game of it to divert your attention away from eating more than you need. Wear a pedometer and aim for five miles a week (then, ultimately five miles a day). Start slowly if you are not used to walking and just add **10** steps more each time you walk—just **10** steps! You may

be surprised how far you will walk. Go ahead and congratulate yourself with every extra step.

3. Read something. This will help to disengage your brain from thinking about food. Notice there is nothing here that encourages you to watch television. Why do you think that is? If you answered because there are commercials that will try to tempt you to buy and ingest high-fat, empty calories, you would be correct. Why spend your hard-earned money and valuable health on what is really "faux food"? Be good to your budget, better to your health, and expand your vocabulary instead of your waistline by reading!

4. Do any household chore. Even if you don't feel like it, just DO SOMETHING—anything other than eat! Remember, your goal is shifting your immediate focus to allow your brain a second to break the thought zone it's in and latch on to another. Just imagine how much cleaner your home will be by accomplishing one chore at a time while losing weight. Now that's time very well spent!

5. Run in place for one minute...rest, then run again...and then again. See how long you can do this. You will be amazed at how quickly you will be able to increase your endurance and your heart rate by doing this for just seconds a day. You don't need to go to a gym or invest in expensive workout equipment. Just stand up and do it! If you don't feel you need to take time out of your day to physically go to another environment to exercise your muscles and move your body, you will be much more apt to do so. This is for your good health, you know, and what could be more beneficial than that?

6   Call a friend. Listen carefully to every word about what is going on in his or her life. Live in the moment. Not only will this help you to refocus your brain, you will be more caring and interested in someone else. It might even help improve his or her day. How many times in our haste do we hear but not really listen? Sure, we are aware someone is speaking to us, but what is that person actually saying? Take the time to involve yourself in your moments. That is all we ever really have; a combination of moments. Envelop your senses in whatever it is you are doing and be cognizant of your surroundings. You control you; your thought processes, your responses, all are within your control. Learning to shift your focus can help in many ways to improve your personal quality of life and reap unexpected rewards.

7.   Clean out a cupboard, closet, or drawer. Take everything off one shelf, or, if you feel particularly ambitious, take everything off all the shelves in a cupboard and really give it a clean sweep. Decluttering is very therapeutic. Ridding yourself of superfluity and "lightening your load" will reflect in the way you feel to lighten your personal load of extra pounds! Shed the clutter—shed the weight! Vacuuming is a good diversion, as it is quite physical and you have to put some effort into it. And see how nice your carpet/floors look afterward—double bonus!

8.   Write a letter or note to a relative or friend. In our fast-paced interactive world, there is a calming aspect to sitting down and putting pen to paper. It seems like an old-fashioned notion, but it actually allows a reflective, contemplative attitude to develop, not to mention a pleasant surprise for the recipient.

9. Brush your teeth, or, at the very least, rinse vigorously with mouthwash. This accomplishes a physical refreshing to your mouth the way refocusing your thoughts does for your mind. It clears your palate like JUST STOP! THINK! clears your mind. Your tongue and taste buds react as if you are finished eating and redirect into a mode of completion. You will not feel hungry.

10. Reread this chapter of the book, or any part you feel is of particular help to you. Remember that this book is like your best friend. It is always there for you, to help you to learn how to help yourself. There are pages left blank for you to keep your own chronological weight-loss journal or just to record your thoughts and feelings, so that when you finish reading this book, you will have your own book full of ideas and responses to what you have read. This way, you can have an ongoing dialogue with yourself, one that will become both self-motivating and certainly self-enlightening, helping to direct you closer to your journey of being what you consider to be your own personal best.

Here's a little bonus suggestion and something new for you to try: put your laundry away one piece at a time. After you fold each piece, put it where it belongs; it burns more calories and gets the job done. It will be effortless in no time, and as long as there are chores to be done, get the most out of them by using more calories at the same time.

This also works for unloading the dishwasher, but you can group like things together: collect all the clean forks, walk over and put them away, then all the knives, etc. This may seem like it takes a lot longer to do, but it really doesn't.

And it gets you moving more, which is the aim; do and move more, not less. You can even make a game out of it; time yourself and try to beat your own record!

Always think to yourself, "How can I best maximize what I am doing to get the most benefit from it?" Soon, it will become second nature to you, and you will be surprised at how many extra calories you will burn by just exerting a little more effort.

Now get going and burn those calories!

MY OWN WORDS

1. What are my thoughts and feelings about what I just read?
2. What will help me "connect" to myself and enhance my mind-body-psyche fulfillment?
3. How can I best use what I just read to my benefit and make it my own?

MY OWN WORDS continued...

MY OWN WORDS continued...

MY OWN WORDS continued...

MY OWN WORDS continued...

Chapter 5
It's Up To You

THINK about the fact that eating one more bite will not bring you closer to your personal goal of weight loss. Really FEEL how you feel. Are you having hunger pangs? Does your stomach feel full? Just STOP and consider this. Do not put another bite in your mouth without really thinking about what you are doing and why you are doing it.

Ask yourself these questions and answer them honestly. Am I eating this because I need to nurture my body and fuel my physical "machine"? Have I eaten a sufficient amount to sustain my life healthfully? Do I really sense emptiness in my stomach? Am I eating because I feel...sad? Lonely? Upset? Dejected? (Or any other adjective or feeling you are feeling.) If you answer yes to any of these, DO NOT put the food into your mouth unless you can do so carefully and with slow determination. Take the time to cut **10** little bites and assess each one. In this way, you are satisfying the need you feel to *have* to eat something, but you are not sabotaging your weight-loss desire and making yourself feel worse in the long run. In executing your personal control, you are giving yourself so much more than one more bite of food can give you. You are giving yourself control of YOU. Your self-esteem will flourish as you attain a positive direction toward your weight-loss goal. You are actually doing something that will improve your disposition, your body, and your life!

Eat only when you are hungry. Don't just eat with your eyes and mouth. Certainly, if something looks good and tastes good it will encourage you to eat, but the way to distinguish if you are really hungry is in how your stomach feels. Feel what "hungry" really feels like so you will have something to base it on. Don't just eat because of the time (breakfast *time*; lunch*time*, dinner*time*, snack *time*). The clock does not know if you actually need to eat something. When you see something that looks delicious, choose when and if you need to eat it. This may seem to be a very basic thing, but it is important for you to discern if you are eating because of genuine hunger, or for any other reason. A taste of something will satisfy you if you are responding only to your mouth and not your stomach. Engage the **10**-bite rule (introduced in chapter 2); thoroughly chew and savor each bite. Having a small bite of something will suffice if you are eating when you are not hungry, but just enticed by something with your eyes and mouth. This "taste" will not only save you from eating unnecessary calories, but will assuage your desire to indulge your senses without engaging your guilt!

It's time to take responsibility for yourself. Put the power into your own hands, your own mind, and your own ability. This is not unattainable. You *can* do it, you *can* attain your goal weight, and you *can* accomplish this! It is absolutely within your realm of reality. No longer is the burden of weight loss an insurmountable challenge. Once you know and practice this, you can apply this philosophy to many aspects of life.

Let's face it: losing weight can be a pain. Who wouldn't want to be able to just *wish* those pounds away? Why does it seem so much easier to gain weight than to lose it? Well, it's time to begin to LIVE-IT, not DI-ET! If you are thinking of how you can get the weight off as easily and quickly as possible, the **10-second** method can certainly help. How much faster than **10 seconds** can it be? It's **10 seconds**: the time it takes to refocus your thinking and really reclaim the control you need to be successful in your weight-loss goals. You can achieve the success you so desire.

The brain is the most powerful organ humans have; there is little dispute about that. So why is it we have a tendency to underestimate the power it has in everything we do? It is time to take back control. Take a few seconds before reacting and before acting upon something. Just THINK. This can be applied to any aspect of life.

We live in an "immediate satisfaction" mind-set. Society has become an enabler *not* to take personal responsibility for ourselves. There seems to be an "out" available for everything, a finger pointing outward instead of at ourselves. It is some "one" or some "thing" else that causes our situation or response. The responsibility lies within ourselves for what we think and ultimately for what we do.

We blame the media for advertising tempting foods for us to purchase. That mouth-watering food is really a photographer's artwork. Most foods you see on television and in print are artificially enhanced. The burgers aren't really steaming (it's dry ice) and the ice cream is really mashed potatoes. (How long do you think ice cream could keep its shape under the hot lights the camera needs for shooting?) In other words, the salability of the product pays off big time to the company making the foods. The better it looks, the better it sells, and the more money for the company's bottom line. But what about your own "bottom line"? Is it getting bigger too?

It's time to really STOP and JUST THINK! Realize that the luscious food you can't wait to run out and eat doesn't actually exist in the way the ads want you to believe. When was the last time anything you ordered, especially in a fast-food restaurant, looked just like the photo? More than likely, you received a flat, paper-wrapped, barely warm item. Just think of all those calories you could save by not eating this poor representation of an edible, healthy-looking meal. It isn't just "fast food"—it's "faux food"! Again, just STOP! Why spend the money, why spend the time, and why spend the calories? With a little forethought and planning, you can eat something healthy, less expensive, and far better for you. There are lots of different flavors of sixty- to one-hundred-calorie yogurt, for example, or you can eat lots of those little carrots and zero-calorie beverages (but water is the best of all for you to drink). Try to find things that are one hundred calories or less. Read every label. Check the ingredients and aim for more natural low-sodium products. That way, if nothing else, you can "bank" calories for a treat if you want one later on. Daily treats are important. Just follow the **10-Second Diet** way:

> Cut it up into **10** pieces and really taste each bite. Chew slowly and deliberately at least **10** times for each bite, really being aware of the aroma, flavor, and texture.

You may find you don't even want all **10** little pieces. When that happens, you know you've really captured the concept and philosophy of the **10-Second Diet**!

It is self-empowering to restrain yourself from eating, even for **10 seconds**. Acknowledge how you feel about having accomplished this. Even if it is only for **10 seconds**, you still did it. Give yourself respect that you can do this.

Do not admonish yourself when you do not succeed in your attempts. Certainly, you may be able not to eat for **10 seconds**, but what about stopping yourself from binging, overeating, or mindless eating? Using some of the techniques discussed in earlier chapters will help divert your attention from the robotic hand-to-mouth action. One of the most important things to remind yourself of is that you need to refocus your attention. Remember that it takes **10 seconds** to redirect your thought process away from what you are doing and change the course in which you are heading; **10 seconds** to successfully transcend from an eating state to a different mind-set; **10 seconds** to give yourself the opportunity to listen to your inner self and at least STOP and THINK of what you truly want to do next. In time this will become second nature. You will find that you won't have to consciously stop for any amount of time. You will be able to naturally stop when you are full and possibly even before that point. You will be able to eat comfortably and sensibly, and retrain your body to eat the amount it requires and no more.

Babies know when to stop eating. They don't binge or require massive amounts of food to satisfy their needs. Through years of exposure to advertising and merchandising we change our outlook, and along with living through more of life's challenging experiences, we seek food as the answer to internal questions. Everywhere we look, from magazines to television, food is there to tempt us. The media tries to convince us that specific foods are a panacea: "Have you recently broken up with a boyfriend/girlfriend? A sugary treat will help you cope." Does this really seem logical?

Eating may be an enjoyment in life, but it is not life itself. And as with so many aspects, moderation is key. Gluttony and eating only for the sake of eating is purposeless. It not only is damaging to the body, but the uncontrollability factor is detrimental to the mind as well. It does not feel good to be out of control. It is emotionally, mentally, and physically beneficial to be in control of oneself. There are so many things in life that are out of our control, at least we can try to control the things we can—and what and how much we put in our mouths is one of these. It is your body, your own self, and only you can control what you choose to put into it. You have the power and control and only you may use it.

Always remember: you have control over YOU!

We may not always have control over what happens to us in life, but we always have control over how we react to what happens to us.

Just say the word NO. If, after that **10**th M&M, you have the urge to shove a handful of them into your mouth, just STOP—say NO! Hearing the word will give you pause to think. Really think about what your impulse is telling you to do. Take a moment to think that all you are about to re-act to is an impulse, a self-destructive pattern that needs to be broken and redirected into a positive, healthy action. Let these thoughts enter your mind. The time it takes to re-think an impulsive response is all the time that's needed to change a repetitive habit. Actually hearing the word NO out loud jars your mind to halt and compels you to listen. Listen to the new and improved YOU! You are the only one who is always with you. You are the one who will change you for the better. You are the only one who *can* change you. Lucky you!!

It doesn't get faster and it doesn't get better than this.

MY OWN WORDS

1. What are my thoughts and feelings about what I just read?
2. What will help me "connect" to myself and enhance my mind-body-psyche fulfillment?
3. How can I best use what I just read to my benefit and make it my own?

MY OWN WORDS continued...

MY OWN WORDS continued...

MY OWN WORDS continued...

Chapter 6
Just Be Nice

We need to develop a more empathetic world. Sympathy is feeling bad for someone. Empathy is feeling *why* another person feels bad. This is not something that will take decades or generations to evolve into. It can start right now. It's time to use your E.Y.E.S.: Engage Your Empathy System. Start thinking and feeling what it would be like to be in someone else's position. We cannot leave it to someone else to try to change our society. It is something each of us must do at every opportunity.

There is too much inconsideration and degradation, too many recriminations and insults. Consider the media and advertising companies that generate this in television and radio commercials, the many television programs and movies produced that show little regard for the respect of individuals. Somehow, it became popular to treat other people in a deprecating way. It has become acceptable to degrade and be insensitive to other people. This needs to stop immediately. There is nothing funny or desirable if you are the object of ridicule. Why should this be a saleable approach to consumerism? Why should companies become bigger profit makers through insensitivity to people's feelings? This approach does not tout the qualities of the product being sold; it only denigrates the competition. As a society paying our hard-earned money, we need to show distain for negative messages in advertising as well as the use of celebrity spokespeople who represent immoral value systems.

Monetary compensation should be commensurate with moral character and ethical behavior. Just because someone is an actor or athlete does not make him or her indispensible in his or her field. The outrageous salaries and media attention are payment enough without the exorbitant amount of money for product endorsements. Look at the behavior that is getting rewarded in many cases. Thanks to good agents and managers, the worse the behavior, the more excusable it becomes. It should not be acceptable and merely brushed off. Many people idolize television, screen, and sports icons and try to emulate their personalities and actions. If they seem to be above reproach, it makes inappropriate behavior acceptable. There should be a responsibility that comes with recognition, and if the behavior is debauchery and disrespect to others, the privileges that accompany such an extravagant lifestyle should be directly affected. In this case, lack of media attention, not being given acting roles, or the revocation of a sport contract would be the biggest penalties. That would send the message that wrong behavior is never the right thing to do. Inappropriate actions do not make one more interesting, desirable, or coveted. Wrong is wrong and right is what must be enforced.

We need to come to a time of individual responsibility, where high-priced legal teams are not enablers to allow so-called celebrities (or anyone else, for that matter) to avoid the responsibility for their wrongdoings. Development of personal fortitude and ownership of inappropriate behavior will help to redefine the parameters of acceptable societal norms. Better yet, just taking **10 seconds** to STOP and THINK before acting in a harmful or disrespectful way before doing anything wrong is the best tactic of all. Here is where the **10-Second Diet** technique works not just in losing weight, but for living a life of the highest quality possible.

People need to be praised and monetarily compensated not for what they can do with a golf ball, baseball, or basketball, but how they treat the people in their life. The same is true for whatever occupation one is in. Once again, it is not what you do for a living that makes you who you are; it is your moral fiber and ethics. These are far more important. How you respect humanity is much more important than how much money you make. Until our society begins to truly admire the depth of individual personal fortitude and care less about physical appearance, we will continue on a shallow path of genuflection to the superficial and not the substantial.

This is not just reflective of individuals, but companies as well. All too often there is a lack of responsibility; a shrugging off of any personal input; a sense of passing the buck, so to speak, so that in the end no one is actually held accountable. Businesses need to substantiate a professional obligation to uphold an ethical and moral foundation to their customers, not just in a monetary sense, but beyond that. The pervasive attitude of "me and only me" has created an insular and egocentric aspect to society. There is a "look at me—aren't I great?" characteristic that is most obtrusive. Reality television has created a genre in which every profession and each daily action is over the top and bombastic. There is nothing "real" about most "reality" television.

We need to contact advertisers and networks and tell them we don't want to see or hear any more insulting or demeaning commercials or shows. We don't need any more debasement in this society. We need to look for, recognize, and celebrate good qualities in others. We need to help other people instead of laughing at their inabilities. This seems so basic and yet it isn't done. We as a society have trivialized the importance of being kind to someone else. The "me" generation is still prevalent. How did putting oneself first in a sentence become acceptable? It is common to hear the phrase "me and you." It should be "you and me." Again, small "bites" of continual consideration will make an immediate and significant difference in someone else's day and eventually in the world.

It isn't a notion that has to be incubated and harvested, the results of which may be appreciated years from now. This is so correct and innate that the effects are felt immediately. It isn't like a law or a mandate, ever evolving, seemingly never culminating, or like a bureaucratic bill that may start out as a good idea, but gets stuck in all the red tape and obstacles until it atrophies into oblivion.

In the animated Disney film *Toy Story*, at one point Woody turns to Sid, the antagonistic character, and says, "Play nice." Well, that's what we all need to do. We not only have to *learn* to play nice, we have to do it. We have to play nice, work nice, think nice, and be nice! We have to start now by taking the initiative to do the right thing, think of other people, and enforce the Golden Rule that the remarkable teacher and humanitarian Hillel stated: Do unto others as you would have them do unto you. Or, a more modern version: Treat others the way you would want to be treated.

After all, how can anyone be "too nice"? (Unless, of course, one is feigning niceness and is actually disingenuous and only out for personal gain at the expense of others. If that is the case, that too has many pertinent psychological implications that go far beyond the surface.) If you are earnest in your attitude and intent on truly being kind and thoughtful, then you cannot be "too nice."

Have you heard the cliché: "Nice guys finish last"? Who decides what "last" is? If you are last in line and the line turns around, then you are first. It's all in the way you look at it. First, last, in the middle, near the front, near the back— it's all relative. Who's to say it isn't better to be that nice "last" guy? There's another cliché: "He (or she) who laughs last, laughs best," which refers more to a revenge situation in which someone gets his or her just rewards. How important is vengeance anyway? It's really all just subjective and rather meaningless in the long run.

While walking down the street in a very nice little city, in an area that prides itself on maintaining an upscale atmosphere and has a highbrow reputation, the man in front of me was eating a confection from a little cellophane bag. He wore a shirt and tie and was carrying a briefcase; it would seem he was a businessman out for a lunch break. When he finished what he was eating, he crumpled the bag into a little ball and just dropped it in the street. I couldn't believe it. In a polite and friendly way I said, "Excuse me, you dropped something." He turned to me and looked mortified, probably not because he was appalled to think he littered, but because he was seen doing it! People may know the right thing to do; if they think they will be noticed and confronted, the chances are good they won't do it. How basic is it not to litter? It almost requires more thought *to* litter than *not* to. You would not consider throwing garbage on your floor and leaving it there; why would you do so somewhere else? Just THINK before you respond or react; JUST THINK about the effect of your actions and rely on your conscience to direct you to do the right thing. If we all acted like we were being watched, maybe we would be better individuals, family members, and citizens in this world.

Regarding the world—to think that world peace is possible at this stage is unrealistic. To imagine that millions or billions of people in the world could all agree on a single premise is improbable when two people under the same roof can't seem to get along, as is reflected in the current divorce rate. Things need to be broken down to the lowest common denominator; not millions of people, just one. A review of history reflects the devastation just one person can do to society. One person can affect so many others in a destructive or constructive way.

It is imperative to act appropriately in our own personal world we share with the people we love, and then reflect that same responsible action in the outside world beyond our immediate family.

The value our society gives to human life seems to be diminishing. When and how did guns and weapons become so prevalent? How did we get so impervious to it? So many innocent lives are lost to impulsive gunfire and explosive anger. There is a *gunsanity* going on and it must stop. This rampant insanity in thinking that using guns for anything one is envious of or finds frustrating is a physical manifestation of seeking power over someone else. It has become a problem of epidemic proportions. Here is a startling statistic: nine billion bullets are bought annually. That is about thirty bullets for every man, woman, and child in this country. ("While Americans usually buy seven billion rounds of ammunition a year, according to the NRA, sales in the past year have jumped to nine billion." CBS Broadcasting Inc. Sept. 24, 2009.)

It is a sad statement that guns have become the weapons of choice to wield power and persuasion without negotiation. The true power we all possess is the impact a creative and compassionate mind can have not just over one person, but used in a productive way to facilitate helpful and life-enhancing qualities to a whole society. We need to advance as a culture from individual physical power over one another in a socially detrimental, devastating way to one that is always moving forward benevolently and altruistically.

Those who feel the need to wield weapons should be pitied, not feared. They need to be reminded that this violence is a symbol of weakness, not strength. Guns and weapons have become as prevalent and acceptable in this society as toys are to children. Looking back in recent history, when was individual violence treated with such nonchalance? Innocent people are victimized while just trying to live their lives. This, above all, needs to be addressed and adamantly dealt with. We cannot just passively allow people to terrorize our neighborhoods and citizens. This needs to stop, regardless of what it takes to accomplish it. We are not barbarians and must elevate and cultivate a higher expectation for humanity, and find a way to live up to it and beyond. This begins by respecting our world and those who live in it. This starts with each individual's acceptance and understanding of being human, which consists of the realization that each of us is created with the three aspects—physical, mental, and psychological—and trying to understand how they influence our existence. Acknowledging and understanding our humanity is not only attainable but mandatory, for without it we cannot fully become a harmonious society, much less fulfilled individuals. It is the goal of living on a higher plane to truly attain a more satisfied and contented life.

There is no shock value anymore. True shock value would be having someone with something valuable to say who can say it with intelligence and class. Vulgarity, profanity, and violence have become passé. There is nothing shocking about these anymore. There was a time when people were horrified by heinous crimes and blatant sexuality, but these have become de rigueur. We need to bring back sophistication and decorum.

Whatever happened to the adage: "If you can't say anything nice about someone, say nothing at all"? Now it seems that all people want to hear is disparaging information regarding both well-known and relatively unknown people. The news and online updates seek out the crude, rude, and lewd daily occurrences on a moment-to-moment basis. Dirty laundry has become something people are proud to share rather than discreetly hide.

It used to be that primarily those who had no better use of the language than to throw around expletives used profanity. Now, the lyrics of songs, the verbiage of comedians, and the casual conversations of people have become littered with one obscenity after another. It becomes a superfluous litany of crudeness that would offend good taste and propriety if only people were cognizant of it. The manner in which one expresses oneself helps define who one is. Words are the vehicles in which we travel through our thoughts in life; without them, we are uncommunicative and misunderstood. It is important to try to explain ourselves as accurately and precisely as possible. In order to do so, an expressive and varied vocabulary is as important to a healthy communication diet for mental and psychological well-being as a variety of fruits, vegetables, starches, proteins, and oils are to a healthy physical diet for the body!

When did being unscrupulous and corrupt become the norm and inappropriateness become acceptable? There are news articles lauding people doing the "right thing" as something out of the ordinary, and unethical behavior has become *acceptable* behavior. Even the way people speak to one another or their children emulates commercials. There is a one-upmanship attitude among people, whether it is between children and parents, co-workers and peers, or just person to person. This smugness and sarcasm is simply rude. Try being the one to apologize first. Say something kind to another person. Be aware that none of us are above anyone else. We are all human beings living life. Refrain from criticizing and critiquing others' appearance or behavior. Just be nice! This attitude can become contagious. If it does not, at least you know that you are doing the right thing. You act civilly and thoughtfully, the way a courteous member of society should act. In this alone, you are improving the quality of your own life and hopefully of the lives of those with whom you interact. Be a positive role model unto yourself and see how much better you feel. Be the person you would like to be like.

When First Lady Nancy Reagan took a stand against drugs, her catchphrase "Just Say NO!" garnered a lot of criticism. It was simple and precise. That's really what it takes. Just don't do it! This can be applied to so many destructive actions. When I met Mrs. Reagan I found her to be a very lovely person and her stance still applies even now.

It seems we are always looking beyond the obvious to make things more difficult than they actually need to be. To bring things down to the basics, the elemental, the simple is often the most effective approach. Why clutter your desk with too many unnecessary papers? Why clutter your mind with too many superfluous words? Life is cluttered enough. It is time to simplify.

MY OWN WORDS

1. What are my thoughts and feelings about what I just read?
2. What will help me "connect" to myself and enhance my mind-body-psyche fulfillment?
3. How can I best use what I just read to my benefit and make it my own?

Chapter 7
Find The Joy

What does it mean to "find the joy"? From the time of this book's inception to now, the economic landscape has undergone a dramatic metamorphosis. Hopefully, the pendulum of society is starting to swing back to a time when people found happiness in the little things. Before the concepts of acquisition and materialism, along with monetary gain, became the be all and end all of our existence. Adding to that is the obsession with "fame for fame's sake," without regard to quality or substance of character. It seems not to matter whether people are thought of as compassionate, generous, or just, as long as the media machine is cranking out their faces on every tabloid or Web site. This personal aggrandizement is superficiality at its very best and is totally meaningless.

Many years ago, a friend of mine who lived in a very affluent area of the country said she went to an estate sale at an extravagant actual estate. She commented to the owner of the house, a woman in her nineties, that there were so many beautiful and expensive things being sold in the house, how could she part with them? The woman said to her, "Honey, I'm going to fill you in on something. You spend half of your life acquiring things and the rest of your life getting rid of them."

How interesting to think that whatever it is we buy, at some point we feel that it would benefit our lives to have it. As if a decorative item, however necessary it seems at the time, actually *improves* the way we live our life.

I am not advocating living life in a barren cave. I am, however, encouraging looking at why we actually feel that an item will affect us in so intrinsic a manner.

In our culture we have been conditioned to believe that more is better. We are led to believe that what you "have" identifies who you are, and the more you have, the more successful a person you are. More is not *better*—more is just more. This is not a beneficial thing when we are "supersizing" greasy, fat-laden French fries or fast foods. This is not of benefit when we consider personal belongings or superfluous "clutter." In both cases, less is more beneficial for our personal health and more important for our own well-being. To put it even more simply: LESS IS MORE!

We need to rethink and reestablish our priorities to ascertain what will truly enhance our existence in this society and our life in general. Getting back to the basics and the essentials in life not only prioritizes what is important, it gives us physical and emotional room to breathe.

The best-seller lists are always full of "successful" self-improvement books. However, they must not be working because people still treat one another with cruelty instead of kindness. The people who could benefit from these books either aren't reading them or aren't following their ideas.

With dieting, as with any other aspect of life, we must learn:

1) Impulse control
2) Frustration management
3) Immediate gratification reversal

Unfortunately, somewhere along the line society has allowed and accepted that one can simply take whatever one wants without regard to another's feelings, thoughts, or well-being. If someone has a whim, it must be met immediately and without regard for others, or even for what is best for oneself. It has become acceptable to obtain material goods or financial rewards through whatever subterfuge one finds useful for the sake of obtaining more things.

As we have already established, happiness or self-ful-fillment may be augmented by the acquisition of material goods, but studies and research have proven that is not the key to true happiness. Certainly, life's basics are essential for a more comfortable existence, but happiness is subjective and may be different for everyone. What truly makes you happy is unique to every individual and must be discovered by self-introspection and honesty. Once again, it is the psychological working with both the mental and physical that will culminate in a clearer understanding of one's self. You simply cannot get away from the "triune diet-y," no matter what aspect of life you are considering!

It has been said that when you are gone, people won't remember what you said to them or what you did for them, but they will always remember the way you made them feel. This is because how you make other people feel affects them personally. It is a personal investment. It is your inter-actions with another human being that become a thread in the woven tapestry of their lives. This is another reason to treat others with courtesy, respect, and kindness.

It is important to listen and respond when someone thinks enough of you to speak to you. My mother told me, "If it was important enough for you to say, it was important enough for me to listen." This is extremely important with the very young and the elderly, as well as all ages in between. Children interact in the world in an innocent and unique way. Truly listen to them, try to understand what they are saying, and let them know you are hearing them. The elderly have lived every day of their lives—a tribute to perseverance. We all know how challenging life can be and to live day in and day out through the trials of life is indeed something worth noting. Their opinions and observations matter; take the time to listen to them. Always acknowledge when someone speaks to you. It doesn't have to be a witty or wise comeback. A simple "I see" or "I understand your point" or even a thoughtful "hmm" is enough to clarify that you are paying attention to them. This interaction between people validates a person's being. It tells them that they do, in fact, matter, and that you are aware of it, which qualifies their presence in the universe. When you speak to someone and the person doesn't respond, do you wonder if he or she heard you? If the person even cares that you are there? Is the person trying to ignore your existence? A simple acknowledgment changes all that, and it is one more step along the path to "Just Be Nice" to others in the world we all share. It makes it just that much more pleasant, at no cost to you whatsoever!

To raise kind and caring children, parents must treat their children kindly and with care. When an adult hits or spanks a child, it is saying to that child, "I am big and you are small." To that parent, life is saying, "I am big and you are small." It is reprehensible to strike a child. Children are small human beings with sensitive feelings. Hurtful words and actions harm the delicate forming psyche. Children must be listened to and respectfully regarded so they in turn will feel as worthy and important as they are. The lessons one learns as a child and these feelings become the foundation of the personal psychological chiaroscuro in the landscape of their lives. People must try to be the parents they would have wanted. You may prove in time not to be the parent your child would have wanted, but you must have someone to base it on somewhere. Truly seeing your parents as the people they are and not what you wanted them to be will help you assess their good and bad characteristics. It is with heartfelt understanding and realization that you can try to get a clearer picture of who your parents actually are. It is from there that you can try to replicate the good qualities and do the opposite with the unfavorable aspects you see or feel. Many things in life offer us the opportunity to absorb and reflect what we feel we want to be, and allow us to bypass and obliterate what we do not want to associate with and what we do not want to be. If nothing else, we establish our preference to be the person we choose to be. We all are products of our own volition.

Those parents who are distraught and frustrated with their disobedient children need to examine their own parenting styles. Little ones need to be taught gently and caringly with nurturing and patient ways. Certainly, a child can and will try one's patience, but this is the time to take a **10-second** mental hiatus and, without physically leaving the child, mentally escape to a calm and relaxing respite. Take a deep breath and refocus on the situation. If it is not a harmful occurrence and the child is fine, reevaluate how you are handling the stress and what you are ultimately teaching the child with your responses and actions. Everything you say and do is a teaching opportunity. Are you reacting with anger and vehemence? What are you telling your child with your actions? Remember, your actions do speak louder than your words.

Keep in mind that the big things in life happen once in a while. Birthdays, anniversaries, births, weddings—all these are pinnacles of emotional (and hopefully happy) times. However, you can turn any day into a special time. Little things happen every day. Embrace and envelop yourself in the small pleasures each day may bring. Keep this attitude in your daily involvements with people you encounter, and with your family, your spouse, and your children. It takes seconds to genuinely look your loved ones in the eye, smile, and say you love them or are proud of them. It takes seconds to write a heartfelt message and enclose it in a briefcase or wallet. A simple note on a napkin in the lunch you made may be just the pick-me-up needed to get through the remainder of the afternoon. Find the time to make others know they are special. Every day offers moments of opportunity to FIND THE JOY.

MY OWN WORDS

1. What are my thoughts and feelings about what I just read?
2. What will help me "connect" to myself and enhance my mind-body-psyche fulfillment?
3. How can I best use what I just read to my benefit and make it my own?

MY OWN WORDS continued...

MY OWN WORDS continued...

MY OWN WORDS continued...

Chapter 8
Be In The Now

NOW is the only time you can live. You cannot live in the past, even a minute ago. You cannot live in the next minute, or even a second later than RIGHT NOW. Therefore, you must focus your attention on the immediate second you are in and really be in it. It is in this way that you can truly live each day to the fullest. Just STOP and LIVE thoroughly in the very second you are in.

You may be wondering how to accomplish this. First, slowly take a deep breath. Begin by concentrating on that breath. Next, really *listen* to your surroundings. Are you out-doors in the vast openness of a forest? Are you in a noisy, crowded office environment? These are two extremes; per-haps you are somewhere in between these two contrasts. Wherever you are, listen to the sounds that surround you. Try to *depict* everything you hear. Usually the word *depict* re-lates to the visual representation; therefore, you will visualize the words you hear. To do so, you need to focus your atten-tion on the sounds. Try to block out what is physically going on around you and concentrate only on the sounds.

Remember, the most powerful and influential aspect of a human being is the mind. Nothing can be accom-plished without it, yet it is the influence of this one aspect that is sometimes least considered. The power of the mind is preeminent for any and all actions, reactions, changes, or improvements to one's life.

In order to be a personally responsible member of society and put it into positive practice daily, here is:

The "Do 10 Nice Things a Day Diet"

Make a conscious effort to do a *minimum* of **10** nice things for others every day. Do as many as you possibly can, but do at least **10**. Most people have at least sixteen waking hours a day. That is a total of 960 minutes, nearly a thousand minutes a day, that you can certainly find time in to exert the effort to do **10** nice things. Make a concerted effort, if you need to, until this becomes effortless. You can and should do as many nice things as possible, but start by intentionally doing **10**. How long does it take to open a door for someone else, or let someone go through the door first as you hold it open? This may sound trivial or inconsequential, but how many times during the day does this happen?

Every day is a clean slate. How will your day look at the end? Will it be cluttered with "I should have...I wish I had...I wish I didn't..." Or will it be full of "I'm glad I did!" How many things in the course of a day do we have control over? How many choices do we make that are all our own? Whatever the number is, when given the opportunity to act or react, decide or defer, do we do so with conscious effort and think about the outcome? Unless it is a life-or-death reaction (which few things really are), how many times do we just STOP and THINK before responding? Try to practice this with little decisions daily, hourly, so that when more important decisions need to be made, you will automatically consider before acting, speaking, or doing.

This may seem pedestrian, almost obvious; however, it is a practice commonly ignored. We can become so involved in our own agenda, the fact that we live in a world with other people becomes obliterated. Don't just stop and smell the roses; really look at them, touch them, and appreciate them! Cultivate appreciation to an art form. Be observant, not oblivious to life and all it offers.

Tell yourself, "Every day, in every way, I'll try to be better and better." Know that you can attain your desire to do so. Look beyond yourself to see how you can help make the world a better place for having been here. Really feel the personal responsibility you have to give back to society. Ponder your unique place in the history of the universe. Self-introspection and innate honesty will help to guide your individual path. It is what not only connects you to your own rightful trail, but to other aspects of humanity. It is the recognition of this responsibility that makes us not only all different in the way we approach our lives, but all the same in the desire to live our lives.

You must learn to be kind to yourself as well as to others. You would no more go up to a dear friend and criticize him or her unmercifully than you would want him or her to criticize you. Don't do it to yourself, either. Don't scold yourself for your past behavior (even seconds ago are in the past). The beauty of life is that it is ongoing. You always have an opportunity to change the way you think and react. It takes just **10 seconds** to refocus and put your thoughts on another track. If you do nothing else, JUST STOP and THINK. All you can live is in the very second you are in. Each second can impact the future, so of course you must always keep that in mind. As you cannot live in the future, you must focus on the **10 seconds** you have now and work on achieving the most positive outcome you can within those seconds. Those **10 seconds** become **10 seconds** more, and so on until you are living in the future you created by living all the **10 seconds** up to now.

To be in command of your time and reactions is self-empowering. You are responsible for your actions and your reactions. You cannot control others. How they react to you and what they say is beyond your ability to modify. However, if you live by exhibiting genuine kindness and thoughtfulness, you may find that you minimize other people's negative responses to you. This is all part of the "just be nice" philosophy. If it seems simplistic that's because it is. Why make life any harder than it already may be?

All too often in life we are made to feel bad about ourselves, either by external factors such as the media's overhyping of the superficial and artificial "beautiful people" (a subjective term), other people's criticism of us, or worse, by our own berating of ourselves for not being like these empty shells we are told are such special people. If "they" epitomize "special," then what are we—unimportant and not special?

You must realize and believe in the fact that every person is special and unique. It is also important to remember that everyone has his or her own thoughts and opinions. All too often there are altercations and raised voices. This is when you need to STOP and THINK. As adamant as you may be about a subject, the other person is just as opinionated and believes his or her position is the right one. When you raise your voice it blocks out avenues of understanding to what other people are saying. It obliterates and shuts down vital communication. It has long been said that if you want to capture someone's attention, whisper. Lower your voice and speak as calmly and clearly as you can, and people will listen. Be sure not to sound patronizing or compliant. How do you best accomplish this? STOP and THINK before you speak! Once again, the most reliable and forthright path to success in dieting and in life!

A country and a society are only as strong as its individual or collective creative thought. Let's delve into this. In a country where promotions and opportunities are based on nepotism instead of genuine creative talent, a wealth of untapped talent and ability never gets recognized. Why? Because someone doesn't know the right someone else. Power and money has taken over kindness and common sense. Popularity does not necessarily equate to wisdom or guidance.

Do not judge people by what job they have. What a person does is not who a person *is*. First of all, do not "judge" at all. Who are we to judge another individual? It is often too easy to make an assessment of someone else by just what we observe. Seeing one small cross-section of someone living an instant in his or her life does not define who the person is. Many circumstances occur that define a person's character. Certainly, if one is engaged in a heinous act it needs to be addressed accordingly. However, too many times individuals are judged by what they wear or by their features. We place far too much emphasis on the physical rather than the true identity of the person, which cannot be seen or assessed in an instant. The qualities a person possesses, his or her disposition, and the unique capability of every human being are not always apparent at first glance. A very attractive and suave individual may have a nefarious nature as his or her true personality. The physical does not always represent the person within.

People are not just the color of their skin, their manner of speaking, or the dollar amount on their paychecks.

What does it take to be a "successful" human being? The makings of a "successful" human being are to accept responsibility for one's actions and create and live a life of personal fortitude with conscience and integrity.

These factors are becoming dying embers in this society. We need to fan the flame of these embers so the fire
doesn't go out altogether. There may at times seem to be a
proportionately small nucleus of people left with this belief
system, but these are the values that will perpetuate the
quality of life.

Conscience. Integrity. Personal fortitude. How would
you define these words? They are not just words; they are
cornerstones, pillars on which to build a "successful" life.
It seems hard to believe that someone can do something
wrong, something to cause misery and pain to another individual, and feel absolved of all wrongdoing by merely ad-
mitting to the act or rationalizing that what he or she did
was acceptable for whatever reason.

Conscience is the differentiating regulator not just to
acknowledge right from wrong, but to encourage right
over wrong. The manner in which one conducts oneself
outside of one's public persona is a testament to the type
of person one really is. Many professional athletes, actors,
and politicians in the news daily personify "people acting
badly." A lucrative career and a high-profile occupation
do not equate to permission to ignore the laws of decency
and consideration. The media enhances and encourages
inappropriate behavior by elaborating upon negative and
repugnant actions, publicizing them anywhere and everywhere, and elevating inappropriate behavior to a level of
social and personal acceptability. This is where personal
integrity needs to be interjected. What is "personal integrity"? Integrity means an adherence to moral and ethical
principles, and to have established a sound character. Personal integrity consists of honesty and conscience. Integrity
reflects a steadfast employment of a strict moral or ethical code. These are personality integers (complete entities)

that lead to virtue and a moral character. All of these are components of being the person you are meant to be, a compassionate and considerate member of society.

Inappropriate behavior is certainly not exclusive to the "rich and famous." Everyday life is full of deceitful and indecent behavior. It is not just a matter of not doing the right thing; it is also a matter of not knowing the right thing to do. There are basic truths going back to the Ten Commandments. There are ways to interact with others on a daily basis that enhance rather than destroy the "human condition." It can really be as easy as: Just Be Nice! Do a nice thing, say a nice word, and behave toward someone else the way you would like to have someone else behave toward you. How simple is this? Life can be hard enough and out of our control in so many ways. Here is a means to have control in a positive and easy way. It is the possibility of briefly brightening a moment for someone else and thus enhancing your own moment as well. It can become a habit simply and easily. Just as uncontrolled negative behavior of some celebrities can be regarded as innocuous after all the media hype surrounding it, having little effect to encourage society's advancement; conversely, small, sincere kindnesses by relatively obscure individuals can make an impact in a constructively beneficial way. One way enhances society; one way does not.

It is imperative to start feeding people's minds and stop feeding people's egos! In Hollywood, they say you have to get through the tinsel to get to the real tinsel underneath. Don't be tinsel—be REAL. Enough of the fame for fame's sake. As William Shakespeare said, "Some are born great, some achieve greatness, and some have greatness thrust upon them." It is not to be interpreted that due to the media and publicity moguls people can be regarded as "great" simply because a gossip magazine puts them on the cover as the greatest, the sexiest, or the best. Why does there have to be a subjective epitome at all? Everyone can be his or her own greatness. One person does not have to be the visual definition of beautiful more than anyone else. The sad thing is that people believe this and feel even more dejected about themselves because they don't think they measure up.

Our current society has an "enough" complex. Why must people feel they are not attractive *enough*, rich *enough*, successful *enough*, or just not *enough*? Who has set the *enough* bar, and why is it set so unattainably high? You are more than *enough* of a human being by just being human, and trying to be the best you can be and make the world a better place for having been here. That alone is more than *enough*. *Enough* of all this other superfluous and superficial nonsense.

MY OWN WORDS

1. What are my thoughts and feelings about what I just read?
2. What will help me "connect" to myself and enhance my mind-body-psyche fulfillment?
3. How can I best use what I just read to my benefit and make it my own?

MY OWN WORDS continued...

Chapter 9
Here's To You

We've had a look at how using the **10-Second Diet** technique can help you not to overeat. Now let's continue to have a look at how that same technique relates to improving the rest of your life.

To STOP, THINK, and wait before reacting is beneficial with the daily tasks of living. Before having an impulsive knee-jerk reaction, if you just STOP and wait, it immediately forces your mind to change focus. Even for just **10 seconds**, it will allow you time to rethink carefully what a better response might be. The term "knee jerk" applies to the involuntary reaction when a doctor taps just below the kneecap and your leg kicks up uncontrollably. This is an immediate and unconscious reaction without contemplation or forethought. So many times we respond to stimuli in this way, and when this concerns something that may affect us adversely, it may create an undesirable outcome.

When you see or smell a favorite food, an initial reaction may be to devour it without considering whether you are actually hungry, or just submitting to the impulse to ingest it. Time for your **10-second** response to kick in: just STOP. THINK. Change your focus and sincerely and carefully consider your alternatives. If you are truly hungry, consider if this is the best selection to satisfy both your hunger and your desire. If you are truly hungry have a piece of whatever it is. Take that piece, not the whole thing, giving you the opportunity to have more if you really want to. Put the piece on a plate—the smaller the plate the better, as the optical illusion makes the piece look bigger. Cut the portion into **10** equal pieces. Look at them, smell them, and finally taste one piece. Thoroughly chew it and enjoy all the aspects of it. Truly taste it. Then, ask yourself if you really want to have another of your **10** pieces. You certainly may eat the other nine pieces, but do so in the same manner in which you ate the first one: slowly, deliberately, and with focused enjoyment on every one of your minimum **10** chews per bite. Again, after each one-tenth portion, STOP and THINK if you really want more. If you can put away the rest of your portion to savor another time, you will feel more in control of yourself. Will it make you feel better to eat or not to eat? It's your choice. Choose what will feel most beneficial to your overall well-being. You have control over you. Did one or two or even five of those small pieces satiate your desire to eat? Just STOP and THINK. Applying this technique to any aspect of life will help you make more thoughtful choices. Being thoughtful and not reactionary when responding to the many decisions life puts in your path will allow you to make clearer and more accurate decisions. Just **10 seconds** of contemplation will help calm you and allow you to refocus and define better outcomes of your actions.

As a society we have developed an "eBay-ization" mentality. In a tenth of a second we see something we want, click a key on the computer, and a purchase immediately satisfies us. But that satisfaction lasts only until the next intriguing item mesmerizes us and we have to have it. So we overpay for something, forget about the fact that there is a shipping fee on top of the purchase price, and don't consider whether or not we need or even want the item in the first place. Acquisition is just so easy. *Having* seems to be more important than actually *needing*. Acquiring more and more—more items, more food—without appreciating it. The attainability of an item more than the desirability is all that motivates the transactions. In seconds the item is ours, whether it's good for us or not.

As we are considering what is good for us, do you know what really being hungry feels like? We do so much mindless eating that we have lost the primal purpose of food. We need to fuel our body when it needs fueling. That is basically it. We've certainly come a long way from that concept. Eating has become an entertainment, a hobby, a livelihood, even a daily goal. It has become a focus of living instead of an aspect of it. Eating sustains us and can be an enjoyable part of life. It should be another aspect of living that gives both comfort and pleasure, in the right proportions. The problem is that eating has become something done in epic proportion, not appropriate proportion. It is time to really look at what part eating plays in your life, so you can understand it and incorporate it appropriately into your daily living.

Science has estimated that hunger pangs last for twenty minutes. Hunger pangs are the biological signal the body uses to indicate that it is in need of an external means of acquiring additional internal energy. An important step in relating to your body is to feel what being hungry is like. If you have not eaten for several hours and feel emptiness in your tummy, then you may experience hunger pangs. If you have eaten a meal within the last hour or so and think you are feeling hungry, just STOP. THINK before you grab something to eat. Get a timer, set it for **10** minutes, and do something else besides eat. Exercise the "**10** Things to Do NOT to Eat" options in chapter 2 of this book. Or, try this: watch the clock. As the minutes sweep by, think about how you are making a thoughtful choice not to impulsively eat.

We all know about the seafood diet: you "see" food... and you eat it! This is habitual, impulsive ingesting. It is not a thoughtful, cognitive response to a necessity in life. During your first **10** minutes of clock watching, use this book as a reference manual and reread your favorite part, the part that is most useful to you personally. Just get through those first **10** minutes.

After that, you will be in the next and last **10**-minute segment of waiting for hunger pangs to subside. Realize that with each passing minute you are one minute closer to fulfilling who you want to be. With each passing moment you are a stronger person. You are a person more in control of yourself, your impulses, your body, your entire being. Every second brings you personal strength. How much faster can you get results than second to second? Just **10 seconds** to feeling better about yourself! As you begin your second and last **10**-minute waiting period, you are at the pinnacle of waiting and the length of time is now declining. The apex of your wait (and "weight") is over and you are sliding effortlessly down the mountain you have scaled. What seemed like a long time to wait for your hunger pangs to subside is now dwindling to **10** more sixty-second revolutions of the second hand, sweeping away your impulse to mindlessly pop something into your mouth. Your twenty minutes are over. Really feel that what you thought were hunger pangs are gone. The emptiness you thought you felt has been replaced by personal fulfillment. You don't feel empty. You feel full of self-attainment. Give yourself credit. If you did not wait the full two **10**-minute segments of waiting time, give yourself credit for the time you did wait. Do not admonish yourself for not doing better; rather, honestly praise yourself for doing the best you could at the time. There's always another **10 seconds** to try again.

You have spent your time well by not giving in to your urge for immediate food gratification. You have begun to break your old self-destructive habit and have replaced it with a new self-empowering habit. This new habit will encourage you and serve you well from now on, for the rest of your life. In addition to the benefits you are already reaping, you are accomplishing this in just **10 seconds!**

Everyone is born with a job in life. Your "job" is to create the best "you" you can be and live that way. Don't ever wish to be someone else; it's impossible and futile. It's just not going to happen. You can, however, try to emulate qualities you admire in another person and cultivate them to make them your own. That will make those qualities unique unto you. Try to be the best "you" you can be. If you are not happy with yourself, take a good look at your attributes and faults, enhance the characteristics you like, and set about changing for the better the ones you don't like. Appreciate all that you have and realize what you may have the capability to be. Give yourself credit for living every day and try to really see the inherent wonder of each one. Remember, do the best you can with yourself, and enjoy who you are, for it is who you are meant to be. Anyway, everyone else is already taken!

Take life **10 seconds** at a time. This is the only time you can exist in, so relish it and try to enjoy it. It goes so fast. Get ready for the next **10 seconds,** for you are already in them.

Does any of this sound familiar:

1) *"I know it's Thursday, but I'll wait until after the weekend to diet. I'll start the week off right; it will help me stick to my diet so I can succeed."*
2) *"It's only a week or two until the new month...I'll begin then, so I can better keep track of my dieting."*
3) *"I'll diet, I will, I'll just do it later on..."*

Well, guess what?

1) Today is your Monday.
2) This is your first of the month.
3) NOW is your later.

Begin immediately—it is time to start. You cannot begin "then" or in the past any more than you can begin "later" or in the future. Take charge of your life and your goals NOW. These are the only **10 seconds** you have in which to begin, so do so. Life is lived neither in the future nor in the past—it is lived now. Remember these powerful **10** words and repeat them to yourself right now:

I CAN DO THIS.
IT WILL WORK!
JUST **STOP**!
THINK!

When you are about to take a bite of something that would be better off not eaten, STOP and say to yourself: "Will this bite bring me closer to my personal goal of how I want to look and feel, or will it make my goal less attainable?" If it will be counterproductive to eat, take the time to THINK about it and put the food down. You will empower yourself with this quick act and it will give you the internal strength you need to continue on your new and successful path to the person you want to be. If you would like to ask yourself the question out loud, do so. Hear the words and respond correctly.

Envision yourself lying in bed at the end of the day after successfully putting into practice this procedure. Imagine how much lighter you feel, how in control you are over your impulse to just pop food into your mouth without a second thought. You have just completed an entire day of moving closer to your personal weight goal. The second day is easier than the first; the third day easier than the second. You have conquered the hold you thought food had over you. You are indeed master of your own will, just like you always have been, but did not know how to really achieve it. Feel proud of yourself; you have learned and accomplished a new and enlightening way to live the rest of your life!

You are in control! You are personally successful and are your own best advocate!

MY OWN WORDS

1. What are my thoughts and feelings about what I just read?
2. What will help me "connect" to myself and enhance my mind-body-psyche fulfillment?
3. How can I best use what I just read to my benefit and make it my own?

MY OWN WORDS continued...

MY OWN WORDS continued...

Chapter 10
Ten Seconds

We are fast approaching page 100. It is a good time to review this book. Look over the pages and reread the passages that are most helpful to you. This is a book to use as a reference and a refresher to keep you steadfast on your journey of life. If you have been writing your thoughts and responses at the end of each chapter, reflect on those. See if your own insights are still pertinent to your thoughts at this time. That is the "you" part of this book. Keep yourself in the "know" and in the NOW. This is the only time you can start to change your life. Begin NOW, the only NOW you will ever have. Enjoy the **10 seconds** you are living. They will be gone and another **10** will take their place, leaving behind only what you have accomplished in that time.

Take a deep breath, take another, and then continue on with your life, doing what you know is right. Within each **10 seconds** try to help make this world, your world, the world you will leave as a legacy a better place. Time is fleeting; life is brief. Make every **10 seconds** count.

You are meant to be the best you can be. How do you do this? By doing the best you can every day. How do you do that? By doing the best you can in every minute, and minutes are comprised of seconds. Do the best you can with every second—every **10 seconds** of every minute, of every day, and you will have a life of fulfillment.

Learning to think beneath the surface involves training yourself to STOP and THINK before impulsively reacting. This is how to elevate the quality of your existence and learn to live a more advanced and fulfilling life. Try to take the brief amount of time it takes to ask yourself, "Why am I doing this?" Answer yourself thoughtfully and honestly. This becomes easier every time you try. Then, you will be able to respond calmly and reasonably without reacting impulsively. You will eventually find that your first response will be one of thoughtful deliberation instead of spontaneity.

Congratulate yourself, as the reward will be in the response. You will begin to understand your motivation, whether it involves your choice of what to eat or in what direction your life will go. With this new response mechanism, you will find that you will make more responsible choices, and ones that will truly guide your path in the direction that will be most beneficial to you.

We have evolved into a *cyber-savvy* society. However, as individual human beings we are, psychologically speaking, predominantly cavemen. Until we learn to incorporate a psychological aspect to everything we think, say, and do, we are stagnant in the area of societal development and human advancement. Realization of the integral impact of the psyche not only existing but being the most pervasive and powerful aspect of our existence is nonnegotiable.

Wherever you look, we are a world concerned with "high tech." However, a society is only as strong as its individual creativity. At the turn of the new millennium, there was a nearly catatonic fear of the "Y2K bug," paralyzing computers and bringing about a technological crash with a Jericho effect. Cyber walls would allegorically be tumbling down, leaving us all in a state of panic. This, of course, did not happen. The real fear should have been that our ability to function creatively would be stultified because it has never been thoroughly explored.

The access is there, the cognizance is not. Until we realize and engage in exploring the vast universe within us, pioneering only the external world is superficial at best. One is not more important than the other. It is essential to recognize and incorporate the fact that they can exist harmoniously.

How do we initially explore the recesses and resources of this mysterious and essential third aspect of our being? Realizing its importance is preliminary. Next, question why you are doing or saying something BEFORE you act or respond. Just STOP yourself from your conditioned I.R.S.—Instant Response Syndrome. Of course, in an emergency situation there are important learned safety responses that should be immediately engaged, but these can be thought about long beforehand and called upon instantly as a survival measure. These occasions fortunately don't arise every day and to thoughtfully and methodically prepare for when they might occur is by all means essential. Apart from those rare instances, very little else in daily life requires a split-second impulsive reaction over one that is carefully and fully thought out.

The time has come to STOP and THINK in life. Learn to really champion the moments of your life every second—every **10 seconds** at a time. Life is fleeting and seems to accelerate with every passing year. Did you ever wonder why the years seemingly go faster as you get older? Why is it that as a child it seems ages until your birthday? To a child, once-a-year occurrences seem so far away. For four-year-olds, a year is fully one-quarter of their lives. What a great percentage that is. With each passing year the gap closes until you are the fulcrum balancing between the years you have existed on earth and the unknown amount of time you have left. We have no time to waste; the years are passing and the seconds are ticking by. The time to delve into your most precious commodity—you—is now.

STOP. THINK of who you really are and why you react the way you do. Compare and contrast that with who you want to be. If you feel you have psychological rigor mortis setting in and cannot answer your own internal questioning at the time, at least STOP and THINK before blurting out words or spontaneously reacting without forethought. By doing this you are at the very least allowing yourself some breathing room to consider your next thought or move. This simple step will produce a level of change. It will allow you to mature and begin to develop your psychological-mindedness.

Begin by realizing something that previously lay dormant beneath the surface and you will start to sow a prolific seed in an otherwise barren emotional garden, one that in time will bloom with understanding of your own motives as well as compassion for those of others. This is the human bond we share; not just that we have a physical shell with far too much emphasis on its superficial aspect; not just that we have a brain with varying degrees of functioning; but that we all have feelings, emotions, and a powerful psychological drive that determines who we are and why we act in the unique and personal way we do. It is this aspect of the human existence that truly makes us the indispensible, irreplaceable person we are. It is this aspect of human life that we cannot replicate or repudiate. This is what truly makes us individual. So why do we not put more emphasis on discovering and cultivating this, instead of all the time, money, and attention that is spent on the genuflection to the physical body—the aspect of humanity that most often degenerates first with the ravages of time? The emphasis needs to be redefined so that kindness and consideration of one human being to another is most important—not how one looks or dresses.

STOP. THINK about this and use the blank page following this chapter to consider your own feelings at this time. Delve deeply and allow your emotions to flourish. Permit yourself to advance in your own personal evolution.

Every day, in every way, you can get better and better. You can gain control of your life in just **10 seconds** at a time.

Before concluding this book, and continuing within the definitive concept of "**10**," here are **10** things you can do to feel better and more realistic about your weight—and life:

1) Don't jump out of bed and onto the scale. You will probably weigh more than if you wait a while and let those sleepy molecules in your body get moving a bit. However, weigh before eating or drinking anything and before you shower; it will reflect a more accurate weight than if you weigh first thing upon arising. Keep in mind that there are days when you have a water weight gain or retention more than other days. Having foods high in sodium, more carbohydrates than you need, or being particularly stressed or tired are all situations that can add to making your body retain fluids. I know that frustrating feeling of thinking you have been "so good" and careful with your food intake, only to find that you haven't lost an ounce and—good heavens!—have even gone up on the scale. Don't worry; it will surprise you one morning with a very pleasant reflection of all your hard work, in the way of a smaller number on the scale.

2) Remember that food is an inanimate object. It doesn't own you; YOU own you. Nothing and no one can dictate to you what might sabotage your diet efforts.

3) Try to understand why you are doing something or eating something. If you are responding to a subconscious deficit of some sort, don't try to compensate with food. It will not and cannot make up for what you feel is lacking in your life. Food fills up your stomach, not your psyche.

4) Do not deprive yourself of something you crave, just don't devour the entire thing. Enjoy the item a little at a time and savor every morsel. You can satiate your desire without ingesting the entire amount. Be cognizant of what and how much you are eating. Make a concerted effort NOT to eat it all. A bit will satisfy your desire. It is only a matter of reconditioning yourself to be satisfied with some rather than all of it.

5) Believe in yourself and the power you possess to accomplish your personal goals, whether in weight loss or fulfillment in life. Know what you want and believe in your innate capability to attain it. If it is to be yours, it WILL be!

6) Realize that other people have the same intensity in their beliefs as you have in yours and respect others' opinions, whether or not you feel the same way. As strongly as you feel, recognize that others feel just as strongly.

7) You cannot be too genuinely kind to anyone else. Treat others the way you would want to be treated. It could not be a simpler mantra, and it is as true today as it always was and always will be.

8) This is the "YOU" you have been given; make the most and best of it. There is not another YOU or another life for you to be YOU. Do it now—do it right!

9)   Think back over the past year. Have you laughed? Have you cried? Were you happy? Were you sad? Did you feel fulfilled, even for a moment? Were you frustrated? Did you sense a feeling of accomplishment, even in the tiniest of ways? Did you love or were you loved, by anyone or anything (a pet, a co-worker, anyone in your life)? A year in your life reflects many moments; some joyous, some not desirable of repeating. Nonetheless, it is a microcosm of your whole life. All of these feelings are expressions of human responses and being alive. Truly, some years may be better or worse than others, but all contain moments of joy and sorrow, fulfillments and frustrations. It is all part of the human condition we regard as life. With this recognition, realize that all things pass, all feelings are capable of changing, and each can be transitional to the next phase.

10) Food is an enjoyable part of life—it is not life itself. There is much to enjoy and experience in life. Get out and enjoy and experience it!

Think of this book like a little one-hundred-calorie (page) confection; however, instead of gaining weight, with every page you learn how to lose weight and gain a better life!

In conclusion, here are **10** simple and easy things to live by:

1)   EVERYTHING IN MODERATION, NOTHING TO EXCESS. Enjoy, indulge, but do so modestly. Eating a lot of something delicious does not make it *more* delicious—it just makes it more! You will not enjoy something decadent more by eating a lot of it. You will just be ingesting more of it and increasing your calories and your weight.

2)   WHEN IN DOUBT, THROW IT OUT! Question the freshness of an item. Certainly, it was fresh when

you bought it; you read the expiration date, if it had one, and thought you would use it rapidly. Somehow, it may have gotten pushed to the back of the refrigerator or cupboard; perhaps you regarded it as something you would "save for later" or you merely forgot about it. After you rediscover it and wonder whether or not to eat it, consider your doubts. If you have even the slightest concern, get rid of it. You won't regret it, and you will maintain your health and safety by not taking a chance on its quality. This logic will save you a lot of stress (and possibly ill health) wondering whether or not you should eat something, and you will feel much better in the long run.

3) IF YOU HAVE NOTHING NICE TO SAY ABOUT SOMEONE, SAY NOTHING AT ALL. Do not lower yourself to disparage or belittle someone else. It will not make you a better person and will only put negativity into your disposition. You really don't know why someone else says something or acts a certain way, so don't assume something derogatory. Keep your attitude elevated and uplifted.

4) TEACH BY EXAMPLE. Hypocrisy does not enhance society. Do not say one thing and then do the opposite. Being the best you can be means listening and learning, not judging and ignoring.

5) JUST BE NICE. It doesn't take a lot of time to be kind to someone. Open a door, say hello, or just give someone a smile. These sound like such benign, simple gestures, yet they are missing so frequently in society. Just start doing thoughtful things and they will become second nature to you, and may improve someone else's day along the way.

6) THINK BEFORE YOU ACT, WAIT BEFORE YOU SPEAK. Words can be weapons. They can hurt and wound. In the intensity of the moment, reacting without forethought can detrimentally change a situation forever. There is a far greater chance that an immediate, thoughtless response will result

in the need for an apology, whereby a considerate, proper, and conscientious reply will result in a more conducive outcome. The former has the greater potential to require retribution, while the latter has more of a possibility to produce a genuine and positive response. Taking responsibility for the human being you are means stopping and thinking before talking or reacting.

7) CALORIES IN—ACTIVITY OUT. There is nothing that will produce successful weight loss other than this equation. The number of calories you consume in relation to the amount of activity you expend will dictate whether or not you lose weight. This is a fact. This is the bottom line. No matter what else you do, no matter what foods you eat, the numbers don't lie and neither will the scale. Of course, the quality of the foods you eat is important. You cannot healthfully survive eating only empty-calorie sweets. However, if you find that you enjoy a "treat" every day, you should have one. Just balance it with the rest of your daily intake and indulge accordingly.

8) FIND YOUR "IT." Find what makes you happy; what motivates you. What is it that you love to do? What would you choose to do all day long, if you could? Is "it" gardening, reading, looking through bookstores, walking, riding your bike, playing a sport, painting, scrapbooking? Whatever captures your attention, gives you a feeling of personal fulfillment, and allows you a mental hiatus is your "it." Seek "it." Find "it." Then, enjoy "it." Focus on your passion and immerse yourself in "it." It is important to create a respite for you to relax and relate to yourself. "It" will set you free to dream, appreciate your desire, and reaffirm your place in life. "It" is your comfort and your enthusiasm in life. "It" is essential to your personal well-being.

9) BE REAL—FEEL. Life is NOT a reality show. Most of those shows are over the top, contrived, and do not reflect how real people act in real life. They are created to garner viewers, not to reflect the "reality" the genre claims to reveal. Don't overreact or overdramatize. Not everything is a life-or-death situation, nor does it need to be regarded with the intensity reflected on television shows or in movies. Keep in mind that if everything is treated with the same degree of importance, nothing has any more or less impact than anything else. Something innocuous would be equal to something essential, and that attitude would prove not to be beneficial. If everything that occurs in the course of your daily living is given the same amount of concern, energy, and consideration—no matter how minute or huge it is—when something really does require your utmost attention it would be on the same level of importance as minutia. In other words, the mail arriving late should not evoke the same level of anxiety as responding to the fact that your dog has run away. There are appropriate levels of emotion that you are capable of regulating. Everything does not need to be nor should be approached with the same intensity. Once again, life is NOT a reality show. Life is showing that you can live "real."

10) THINK FOR YOURSELF. Don't do what others are doing simply because they are doing it. Do not emulate "celebrities acting badly," doing illegal or immoral things. Never forget you are a person—not a persona. Try to do what you can to elevate the moral state of humanity. Let your own conscience guide your actions and listen to your inner instincts, as they can generally be trusted to guide your motivations into right rather than wrongful actions. This is how to engage the mind-body-psychological oneness that a human being must strive to attain for true fulfillment. Be the

shepherd, not the sheep. Be the leader, not the follower. Don't buy something just because someone you recognize is being paid to sell it to you. Why spend your hard-earned money on some product that a well-known person is endorsing? It does not validate the quality of the item nor enhance its ability to perform beyond expectations just because a celebrity or sports icon is touting it. Think for yourself. Be yourself. Don't be someone or something you are not. You are the only, original, and unique "you" there is—make it the best "you" possible.

Remember these **10** simple words:

I CAN DO THIS.
IT WILL WORK!
JUST **STOP**!
THINK

Focus on the moment you are living in to make it the best you can, and enjoy your life in a new and enlightened way beginning now—in these **10 seconds**!

MY OWN WORDS

1. What are my thoughts and feelings about what I just read?
2. What will help me "connect" to myself and enhance my mind-body-psyche fulfillment?
3. How can I best use what I just read to my benefit and make it my own?

THE 10-SECOND DIET

Reference Guide

Here is a quick reference guide so you can easily locate the chapter you would like to reread for an additional motivational boost whenever you need it.

Chapter 1
You Can Do It

This chapter gives an overview of what you will begin to uncover about your own motivation regarding dieting and food selections. It gives you immediate empowering of your own will to accomplish your goal.

Chapter 2
Stop & Think

One of the basic concepts of THE 10-SECOND DIET is not to react immediately, and to control the basic urge to just respond, whether to food or impulses in life. There is a unique and easy technique to be mastered and this chapter presents it, along with the methods to achieve success.

Chapter 3
Keep It Easy

So many times, the simplest of tasks can become difficult by overthinking or overdoing. This chapter clearly and easily defines the procedures and thought processes to attain your goals readily and without any additional self-imposed obstacles. The lessons in this chapter may be used immediately to begin the personal uncluttering of your life.

Chapter 4
Keep Moving

The slightest actions are better than just sitting still. Here, THE 10-SECOND DIET explains how to "keep moving," and inspires both physical and mental activity to continually move forward to reach your weight-loss goals. This same philosophy is also used in accomplishing your lifelong or even daily personal ambitions.

Chapter 5
It's Up To You

The ability of this chapter to motivate and empower you results in a healthier and happier way to approach life and living. We are capable of seizing the seconds in life and doing the best we can with them. Many times we victimize ourselves without realizing it. This chapter gives an instant new outlook, along with exercises to stimulate and revitalize your thought processes. It's not a matter of what other people can do *for* or *to* us; it is how we respond to what happens to us. To modify the way we think is essential to progress and develop new attitudes that will enhance our lives. The power to improve and ultimately change really is up to you.

Chapter 6
Just Be Nice

Such an innocuous title and so easy to do, yet we encounter negative instances every day that could be alleviated by putting this into practice. Here is where THE 10-SEC-

OND DIET really begins to assess societal conscience and brings awareness to how we interact with others. The simplest of acts may bring about the biggest of changes. This chapter is an eye-opener that can help you reassess your own behavior and reactions to others, and see the positive difference each of us can make.

Chapter 7
Find The Joy

Sometimes, the very things we seek the most are there before us, hiding out in the open. When we feel badly about ourselves, we can be our own worst enemy. We may have a tendency to denigrate our feelings before we think others will criticize, belittle or malign us. It is easy to forget the important things. This is when we need to look for and discover even the slightest of the good that is all around us.

Chapter 8
Be In The Now

The one thing we have is the second we are living right now. We cannot live in the future or relive the past. It is essential to be submersed in the seconds you are living as fully as possible. This chapter reveals how to accomplish this, as well as how this is the key to success in both dieting and living.

Chapter 9
Here's To You

This chapter champions reconsidering your thoughts about yourself and the changes you feel you need to make. THE 10-SECOND DIET neither condemns nor condones the life you live; it encourages a new way to live your life, starting immediately. This is common sense, and instead of pointing out what you may have done wrong in the past, it urges you to begin refocusing your thoughts to fulfill your own personal goals and feel a sense of accomplishment instantly.

Chapter 10
Ten Seconds

This chapter reiterates the technique described throughout the book. It is essential to elaborate upon and encourage the value of the very life you live **10** seconds at a time. Changes can be made in just **10** seconds and THE 10-SECOND DIET shows you how. Mastering this simple technique can change and improve your life.

Made in the USA
Charleston, SC
12 April 2014